Ines KAMMOUN
Sana SELLAMI

GUILLAIN BARRE SYNDROME

Ines KAMMOUN
Sana SELLAMI

GUILLAIN BARRE SYNDROME

From physiopathology to electroneuromyographic exploration

ScienciaScripts

Imprint

Any brand names and product names mentioned in this book are subject to trademark, brand or patent protection and are trademarks or registered trademarks of their respective holders. The use of brand names, product names, common names, trade names, product descriptions etc. even without a particular marking in this work is in no way to be construed to mean that such names may be regarded as unrestricted in respect of trademark and brand protection legislation and could thus be used by anyone.

Cover image: www.ingimage.com

This book is a translation from the original published under ISBN 978-620-3-45053-8.

Publisher:
Sciencia Scripts
is a trademark of
Dodo Books Indian Ocean Ltd. and OmniScriptum S.R.L publishing group

120 High Road, East Finchley, London, N2 9ED, United Kingdom
Str. Armeneasca 28/1, office 1, Chisinau MD-2012, Republic of Moldova, Europe
Printed at: see last page
ISBN: 978-620-5-70232-1

Dr. Ines KAMMOUN: Associate Professor in Physiology and Functional Explorations

Dr. SanaSELLAMI : Resident in physiology and functional explorations

PLAN

CHAPTER 1: THE BASICS OF NEUROPHYSIOLOGY APPLIED TO THE CLINIC

The brain is considered the foundation of the soul, the mysterious source of those mental peculiarities, which we believe set man apart from animals. The brain and the spinal cord are also **centers of integration of homeostasis, movement** and many **other functions**. They are the control centers of the nervous system, a network of billions of nerve cells linked together in a highly organized way to ensure rapid control of the body. Nerve cells, or **neurons**, are designed to carry electrical signals quickly and, in some cases, over long distances. Their structure is exceptional and many have long, thin extensions, which can stretch more than a meter long. In most pathways, neurons release chemical signals, called **neurotransmitters**, into the extracellular fluid. In a few pathways, neurons are connected by gap junctions that allow electrical signals to pass directly from one cell to another. What is exceptional about the nervous system is the sophistication of the organization of interconnection networks. Reflex pathways do not necessarily follow a straight line from one neuron to another(1).

1. ORGANIZATION OF THE NERVOUS SYSTEM

The nervous system is structured into the CNS including the brain and spinal cord and the PNS (Figure 1). The role of the PNS is to transmit information between the CNS and the rest of the body. It is made up of:

• peripheral receptors sensitive to a type of sensory modality (touch, taste, etc.)
• afferent pathways that carry information translated into electrical signals from peripheral receptors to the CNS.

• efferent pathways that carry the information translated into electrical signals from the CNS to the peripheral effector organ, which thus ensures the answer. They are of two types: the efferent part of the somatic nervous system which innervates the skeletal muscles and whose neurons are called motor neurons or motor neurons for this reason and the efferent part of the vegetative nervous system which innervates the smooth muscles, the cardiac muscle, the glands and the digestive tract(1).The CNS is made up of integrating centers that process, organize and respond to information. The information is transmitted by the interneurons(2)

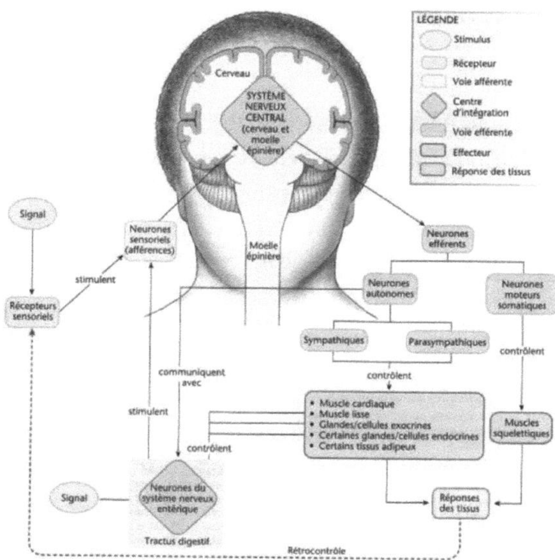

Figure 1: Organization of the nervous system

The flow of information through the nervous system follows the basic reflex modality.Sensory receptors distributed throughout the body continuously monitor the conditions of the external and internal environments. These receptors send information along afferent neurons to the CNS. The CNS is the integration center of the nervous reflexes (figure 2). Its neurons integrate the information that arrives through the afferent branches of the PNS and determine the need for a response.

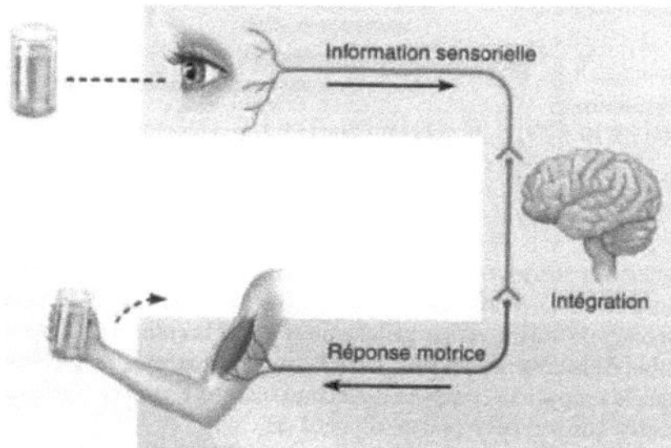

Figure 2: Functions of the nervous system: Example: a thirsty person who sees a glass of water and grabs it

The CNS emits signals that induce an appropriate response, which migrates through the efferent neurons to the effector cells of the body. Efferent neurons are classified into **a somatomotor group**, which controls skeletal muscle, and an **autonomic group**, which controls smooth and cardiac muscle, exocrine glands, some endocrine glands, and some types of fatty tissue. The autonomic nervous system group of the PNS is also called the visceral nervous system (VNS) because it controls contraction and secretion within various organs [visceres, internal organs]. The neurons of the autonomic system are further subdivided into **sympathetic and parasympathetic** systems, which are distinguished by their difference in anatomical organization and the substances they use to activate target cells(3). Very recently, a third group of the nervous system has received special attention. This is the enteric nervous system (ENS), which is a network of neurons located in the wall of the digestive tract. It is often solicited by the ENS, but has the ability to function autonomously through its own integration center. The role of neural reflexes is essential in the communication, coordination and homeostasis of the body, it should be noted that important mechanisms can take place in the CNS without the intervention of inputs or outputs of the PNS(1).

1.1. **Peripheral nervous system**

The PNS is made up of nerves. A nerve is a collection of several nerve fibers (neurons) that travel together to the same destination. The grouping of cell bodies in the PNS is called a ganglion. There are four types of ganglia: spinal, sympathetic, parasympathetic and enteric (digestive). By abuse of language, a distinction is made between myelinated or amyelinated nerves. In fact, it is the nerve fiber, the unitary element of the nerve, that is myelinated or not. Thus, a nerve is an assembly of nerve fibers of different constitution. The nerve fibers are the axons of afferent neurons and the axons of efferent neurons. The afferent neuron has the particularity of not having dendrites but a single axonal extension. From the cell body an extension is emitted to the central nervous system. The efferent neuron has many dendrites and a single axonal extension to its effector(4).

1.2. Central nervous system

The CNS includes the brain protected by the cranium and the spinal cord, a cylinder of nervous system protected by the spine (Figure 3) (5).

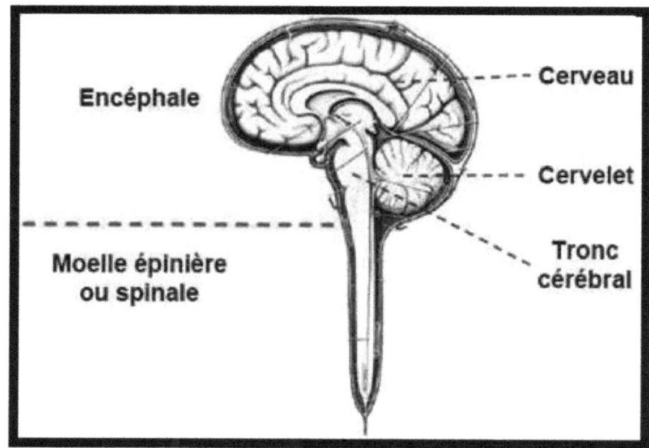

Figure 3: Central nervous system (Nevraxe)

The meninges consist of three layers that lie between the bone and the CNS; the dura mater abuts the bone, the piala mater abuts the nervous tissue, and the arachnoid lies between the two (Figure 4).

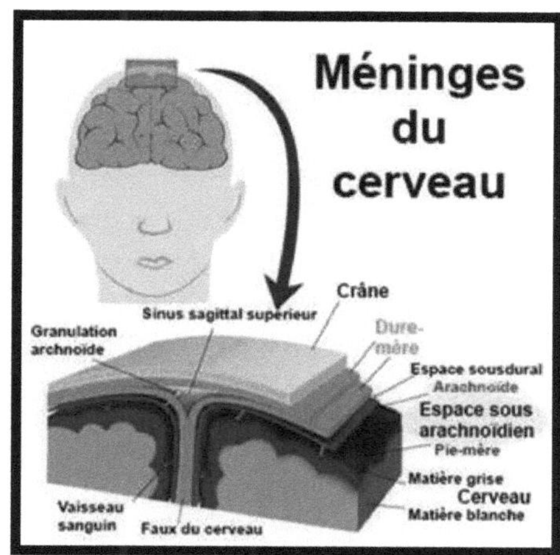

Figure 4: The meninges of the brain

The subarachnoid space is defined as the space between the pie-mother and the arachnoid;it contains the fluid cerebrospinal fluid (CSF) or fluid

The cerebrospinal fluid (CSF) has many roles, including that of a mechanical buffer between the nervous tissue and the bone(6).

1.2.1. **Spinal Cord:**

It has 3 functions
• it is the receiving and effector center of each metameric level of the body, materialized by the sensory and motor nerves
• it is the first integrating center of the nervous message by its transverse circuits
• it is a conduction pathway for nerve messages: it is crossed longitudinally by **bundles of** descending **axons** that transmit motor information from the brain to the spinal cord, and by bundles of ascending axons that transmit sensory information to the brain.

On a cross-section, the gray matter (GM) is visible in the center and is shaped like a butterfly. Surrounding the gray matter is the white matter (WM), which consists of myelinated axons(5). The mediodorsal or posterior septum and the medioventral or anterior sulcus distinguish two hemimoels of identical anatomy and function(7).

1.2.1.1. **White substance**

White matter axon bundles are grouped into three pairs of cords that run from back to front:

• the posterior cords
They transmit the deep conscious sensitivity (sense of position of a body segment in space) and the epicritic tact (fine or discriminative tact): they are exclusively ascending;
• the lateral cords located between the dorsal (posterior) and ventral (anterior) roots have ascending pathways transmitting the Painful and thermal sensitivity in particular, and descending (crossed pyramidal bundle);
• the anterior cords are made up of descending motor pathways (direct pyramidal bundle and extrapyramidal tecto-, vestibulo-, olivo- and rubrospinal bundles) and ascending ones.

Thus, these anatomical bundles correspond to a different functionality.

1.2.1.2. **Grey matter**

The gray matter is organized in horns.
• The posterior horns receive fibers from the posterior roots and serve as a relay for thermoalgesic sensitivity (thermal and painful sensitivity).
• From the lateral horns emerge sympathetic preganglionic fibers from D1 to L2 and parasympathetic preganglionic fibers from S2 to S4 providing a vegetative function.
• From the anterior horns, neurons originate from the anterior roots and descend from the entire nervous system. They receive sensory information from peripheral receptors either **directly from the** dorsal **roots or indirectly through intersegmental association pathways** of neurons from the contralateral posterior horn (Figure 5).

The neurons from the anterior horns are the motor neurons that innervate the extrafusorial skeletal muscle fibers responsible for movement.

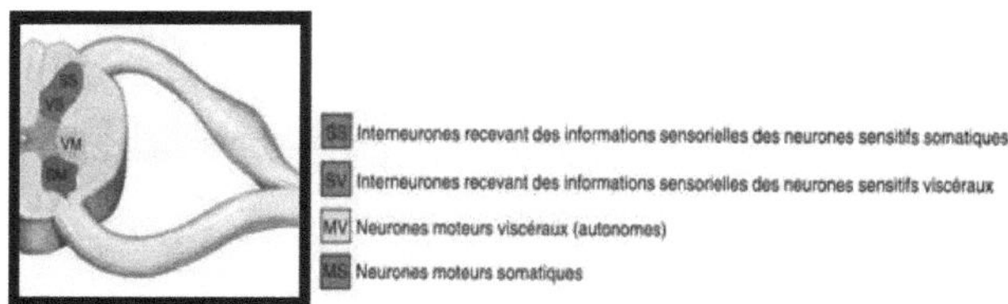

Figure 5: Organization of the gray matter of the spinal cord

At each level of the spinal cord, we recognize a ventral (or anterior) root and a dorsal (or posterior) root that carries the spinal ganglion, the seat of the cell bodies of the sensory neurons. At the level of the spinal foramen, the two roots join to form the spinal nerve.There are **31 pairs of spinal nerves**; 8 pairs of cervical nerves, 12 of thoracic nerves, 5 of lumbar nerves, 5 of sacral nerves and 1 of coccygeal nerves. The spinal nerves are mixed nerves (consisting of sensory and motor fibers) that are connected to the spinal cord by a dorsal (posterior) sensory root and a ventral (anterior) root. Shortly after its emergence, this nerve gives rise to a dorsal branch that innervates the paravertebral muscles. The ventral branch of these nerves takes charge of a different body segment or **metamerium** depending on the anatomical level from which it arises (Figure 6). At the thoracic level, these nerves remain individualized. At the cervical, lumbar and sacral levels, the spinal nerves exchange fibers with each other forming a network or nerve plexus called the brachial plexus and lumbosacral plexus. From this network, the sensory-motor nerve trunks emerge. The roots, plexuses and nerve trunks define the PNS.

-The body territory innervated by a single dorsal root is called **dermatome**: this is a sensory territory
-The body territory innervated by a single ventral root is called **myotoma**: this is a motor territory(7).

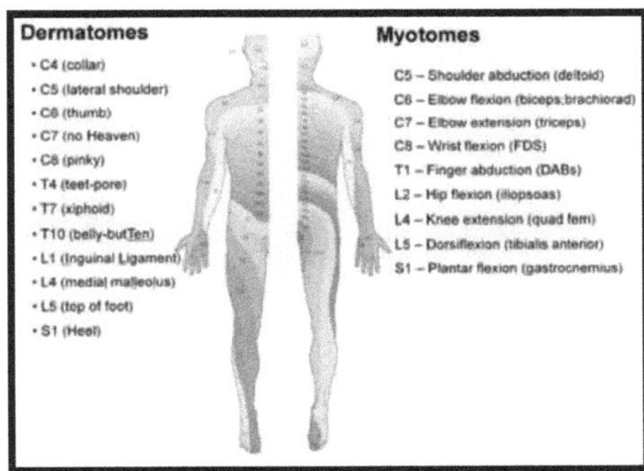

Figure 6: Body innervation in metameres: Dermatomes and Myotomes

One of the particularities of spinal nerves (Figure 7) is that they are all mixed, i.e. **they all contain afferent and efferent neurons.**

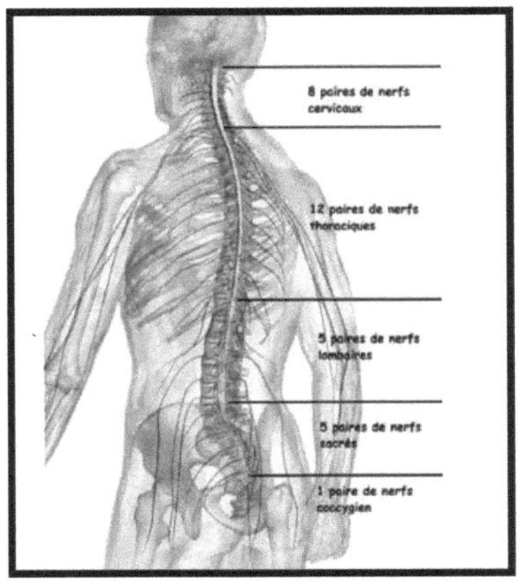

Figure 7: Schematic representation of the 31 pairs of spinal nerves.

Depending on whether or not the effectors of the peripheral nervous system are voluntarily controllable, it is subdivided into :

- **somatic nervous system**
- **vegetative or autonomic nervous system.**

Indeed, while the efferences of the somatic nervous system innervate only the striated skeletal muscles, those of the vegetative nervous system innervate the smooth muscles, the cardiac muscle, the endocrine and exocrine glands, the enteric nervous system as well as part of the adipose tissue (figure 8)

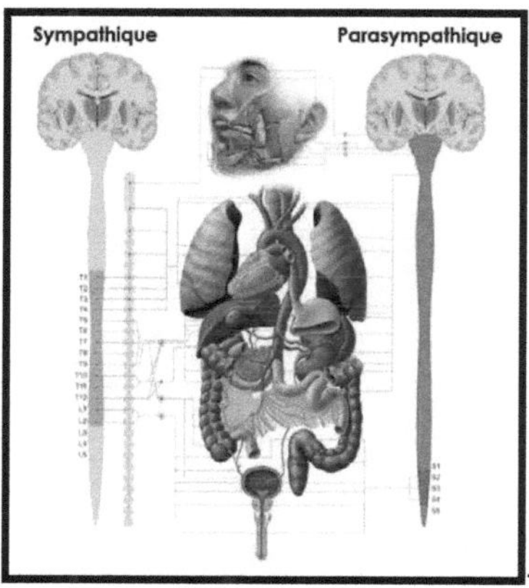

Figure 8: representation of the central origin of the vegetative nervous system (sympathetic and parasympathetic)

The afferent pathways of the peripheral somatic and vegetative nervous system are direct, without relay. The neurons, of unipolar type, have their cell bodies located in the spinal ganglia for the spinal nerves or in the sensory ganglia of the cranial nerves (Figure 9).

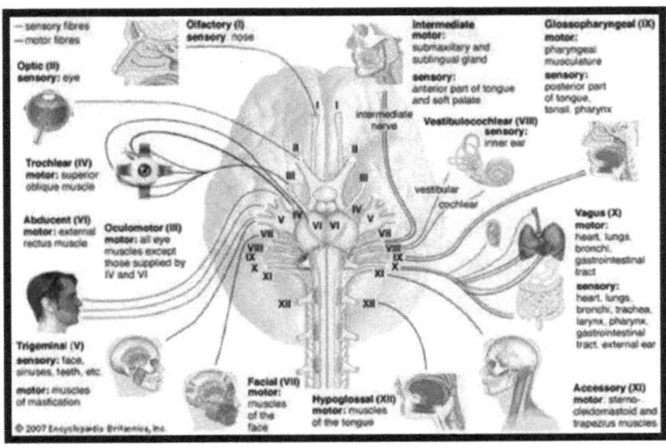

Figure 9: The twelve pairs of cranial nerves

When the afferent is a spinal nerve, it enters the spinal cord through the dorsal root.The efferent pathways of the somatic nervous system, which control the striated skeletal muscles, are direct.

The cell bodies of the neurons are located :
• or in the brain,
• or in the anterior horn of the spinal cord.
From the cell bodies, the axons, myelinated of type α, go directly to the striated skeletal muscle without any relay by leaving the central nervous system :

• or through the ventral root of the spinal cord,
• or through a foramen for the cranial nerves.
These axons can therefore be more than 1 meter long for those that innervate, for example, the foot muscles.

At the effector level, the axon synapses on several muscle cells forming the muscle junction. Thus, a single neuron controls several muscle fibers at the same time (the set formed by the neuron and the muscle fibers it controls defines the motor unit).The neurotransmitter released at the neuromuscular junction by somatic efferent axons is acetylcholine. This binds to nicotinic receptors on the muscle cell membrane.The nicotinic receptor is an ionotropic receptor which, when it has attached two acetylcholine molecules, opens and lets sodium into the cell.The muscle cell thus undergoes depolarization which, if sufficient, causes an action potential triggering contraction of the muscle cell with a purely excitatory influence on striated skeletal muscles (Figure 10).

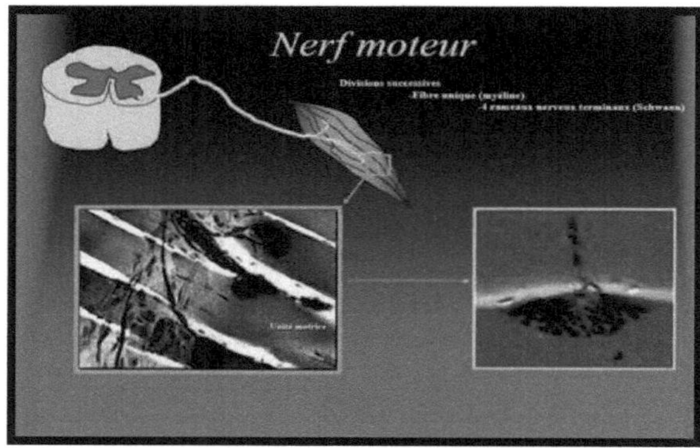

Figure 10: Schematic representation of the organization of somatic efferent pathways

2. CLASSIFICATION OF REFLEX PATHWAYS

A reflex arc requires five elements.
- **Receptor.** Dendritic terminals of a sensory neuron, located in the skin, in a tendon or joint, or located in other peripheral organs, that respond to specific stimuli.
- **The sensory neuron.** Starts from the receptor and passes through the dorsal root to bring the sensory impulses to the dorsal horn of the spinal cord.
- **The nerve center.** Grey matter of the spinal cord where sensory and motor neurons are articulated slowly or via one or more interneurons.
- **The motor neuron.** Conducts nerve impulses from the ventral horn of the spinal cord, through the ventral root, to the effector organ.
- **The effector.** The muscle that responds to the motor impulse by contraction or the gland that responds to this impulse by secretion.

Reflex pathways in the nervous system are composed of chain-like networks of neurons, which connect sensory receptors to muscles or glands. Reflex pathways can be classified in different ways (Table I):

1. By an efferent division of the nervous system that controls the response. Reflexes that involve somatomotor neurons and skeletal muscles are called **somatic reflexes**. Reflexes that are controlled by vegetative neurons (Figure 11) are called **vegetative reflexes**.

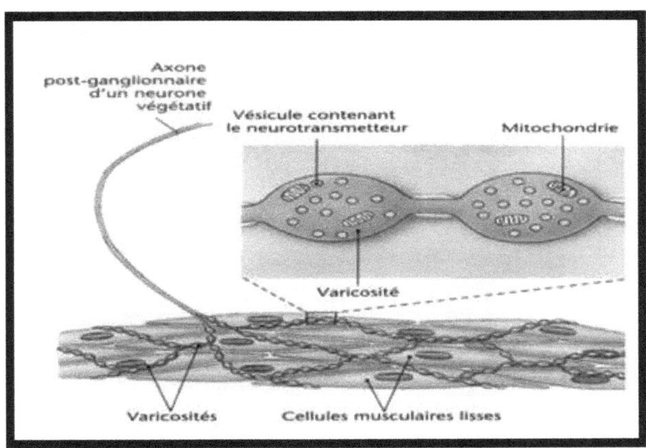

Figure 11: **Varicosities of vegetative neurons that control a smooth muscle**

2. By the location of the CNS where the reflex is integrated. **Spinal reflexes are** integrated in the spinal cord. These reflexes can be modulated or not by signal inputs from the higher brain. Reflexes integrated in the brain are called **cranial reflexes**.

3. By whether the reflex is innate or acquired. Many reflexes are **innate**, which means that we are born with them and they are genetically determined. An example is the patellar (or tendon) reflex, in which the lower leg tightens when the patellar tendon on the upper part of the patella is stimulated (kicked or pushed). Other reflexes are acquired through experience.

***The example of Pavlov's dog salivating when he hears a bell ring is a classic acquired reflex, also called a conditioned reflex.

4. By the number of neurons involved in the reflex pathway. The simplest reflex pathway is represented by the **monosynaptic reflex**, whose name comes from the fact that there is only one synapse between the two neurons of the pathway: a sensory afferent neuron and a somato-motor efferent neuron (figure 12).

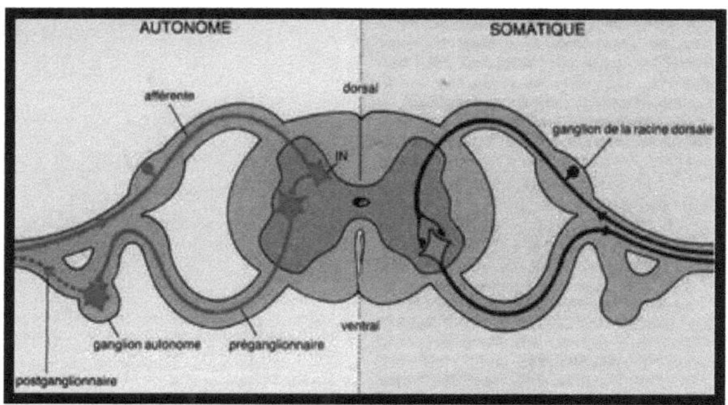

Figure 12: General organization: comparison of autonomous reflex arc and somatic reflex arc; IN interneuron

Table I: Nerve reflexes can be classified according to :

1.*The efferent division that controls the effector*
a. *Somatomotor neurons control skeletal muscles.*
b. *Vegetative neurons control smooth and cardiac muscles, glands and adipose tissue.*

2.*The region of integration in the central nervous system*
a. *Spinal reflexes do not require input from the brain.*

b. *Cranial reflexes are integrated in the brain.*
3.*The time during which the reflex develops*
a. *Innate reflexes are genetically determined.*
b. *The acquired (conditioned) reflexes are acquired by experience.*
4.*The number of neurons in the reflex loop*
a. *Monosynaptic reflexes have two neurons: an afferent neuron and an efferent neuron. Only somatomotor reflexes can be monosynaptic.*
b. *Polysynaptic reflexes involve one or more interneurons between the efferent and afferent neurons. All vegetative reflexes are polysynaptic because they have three neurons: one efferent and two afferent neurons.*

CHAPTER 2: PATHOPHYSIOLOGY OF GUILLAIN-BARRE SYNDROME

Guillain-Barré syndrome (GBS) is an autoimmune poly-radiculoneuropathy of acute onset(8, 9). It is a clinical entity characterized by the rapid onset of symmetrical limb paralysis, tendon areflexia, absent or minor sensory disturbances and variable autonomic nervous system involvement (cardiac arrhythmia, blood pressure dysregulation, ileus, urinary disorder)(10-12). It is the most frequent cause of acute paralysis in the world (13, 14). This syndrome evolves in 3 phases (Figure 13): an ascending phase lasting up to 4 weeks, a plateau phase and a recovery phase(15, 16).

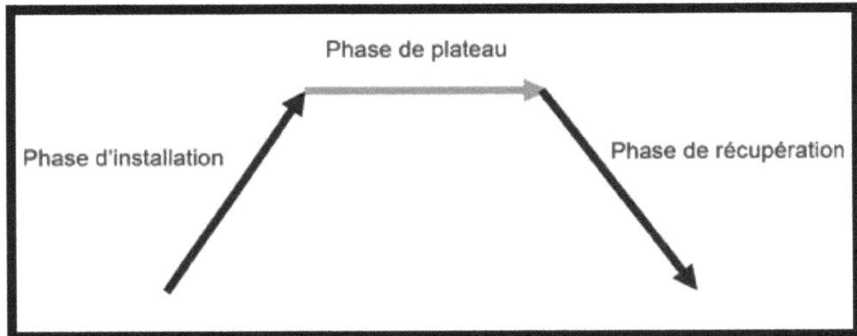

Figure 13: The evolution of Guillain-Barré syndrome

Biologically, it is characterized by the presence of a dissociation albumino-cytological in the cerebrospinal fluid.The pathophysiological mechanisms and clinical presentations of GBS are variable(17-19). The clinical spectrum of GBS is dominated by the classic form characterized by weakness of the 4 limbs, most often ascending, with osteotendinous areflexia, which may or may not be associated with cranial nerve damage or dysautonomic signs.In addition to this classical form, other related or focal forms of GBS have been reported(20, 21). GBS can occur at any age but is rare in childhood(22).

There are several variants of GBS:

• Sensory-motor: acute inflammatory demyelinating polyradiculoneuritis (AIDP; the most common) or acute axonal sensory-motor neuropathy (AMSAN).

• Pure motor: acute demyelinating motor neuropathy (AMD) or acute motor axonal neuropathy (AMAN)(23)

• Miller-Fisher syndrome: ophthalmoplegia, ataxia and areflexia

• Bickerstaff brainstem encephalitis (BE): similar to Miller-Fisher syndrome, but also includes altered consciousness (encephalopathy) and/or hyperreflexia (24, 25).
• Pharyngo-cervico-brachial form: acute weakness of the arm, impaired swallowing and weakness of the facial muscles (26).
• Acute pandysautonomia: diarrhea, vomiting, dizziness, abdominal pain, ileus, orthostatic hypotension and urinary retention, bilateral tonic pupils, fluctuating heart rate, decreased sweating, salivation and lacrimation (27).

• Pure sensory: acute sensory loss, sensory ataxia and areflexia but no motor impairment (26, 28).
It is difficult to distinguish the 3 main forms of GBS (Figure 14): AIDP, MAN, and AMSAN on the basis of clinical signs.

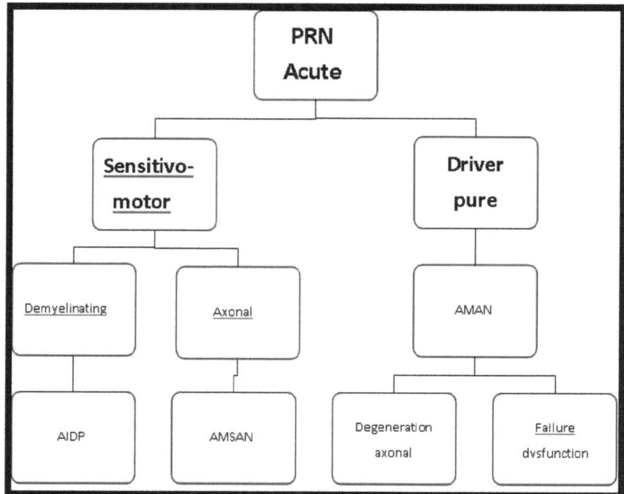

Figure 14: The different forms of acute polyradiculoneuritis

Pathophysiologically, AIDP is due to an aberrant cross immune response. Indeed, there is a phenomenon of molecular mimicry between the antigens of certain bacterial or viral liposaccharides and certain constituents of peripheral myelin.Macrophages activated by the immune reaction attack the surface antigens of the myelin sheaths, resulting in segmental demyelination, which leads to blockage or slowing of nerve conduction and clinically to flaccid paralysis. In some severe and prolonged forms, demyelination may occur accompanied by secondary axonal degeneration. The latter may lead to misclassification as axonal. In the primary axonal forms of GBS (AMAN, AMSAN), there is a nodal and paranodal involvement secondary to an attack by antibodies antigangliosides. IgG antibodies bind to GM1 or GD1a gangliosides present on the axon at the nodes of Ranvier and cause the disappearance of voltage-gated sodium channel clusters. Nodal and para-nodal changes disrupt nerve conduction and lead to axonal degeneration. Demyelination and lymphatic infiltration are minimal (29). In experimental models and in AMANs it has been shown that antiganglioside antibodies attack not only the nodes of Ranvier but also the paranodal regions and cause detachment of myelin from the paranodal regions mimicking paranodal demyelination (Figure 15). This could explain the presence of antiganglioside antibodies in patients meeting the criteria for demyelination.

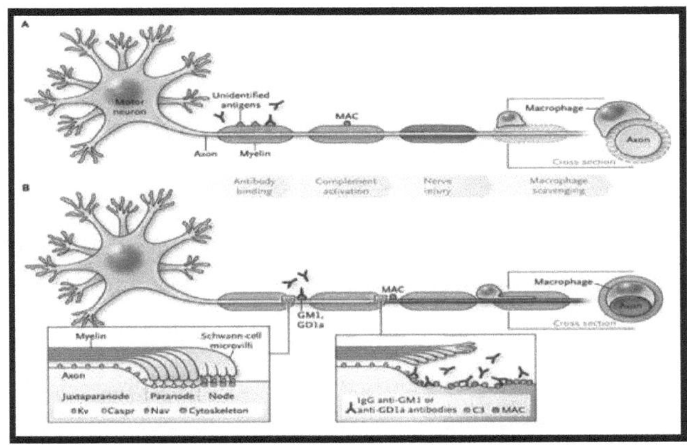

**Figure 15: Pathophysiological mechanisms of the demyelinating form (A)
and the axonal form (B)(30)**

AIDP patients have a longer duration of the extension phase than patients with AMAN(31).Antiganglioside antibodies are more frequently found in axonal forms; their presence in AIDP has been debated at length (32, 33). In recent Italian and Japanese series, antiganglioside antibodies were found in all patients reclassified as axonal (AIDP or equivocal). An even more recent study showed that in AIDP, inflammatory infiltrates containing T cells and macrophages are present, with macrophages involved in myelin removal. Antibodies and membrane attack complexes can also be detected on Schwann cells.

Furthermore, in AIDP, segmental demyelination and subsequent remyelination result in progressively slower nerve conduction velocities, prolonged distal latencies and temporal dispersion (13).AMAN is primarily antibody-mediated, with IgG and activated complement proteins. Macrophages contribute to axonal injury by invading the periaxonal space between the axon and myelin. The antibodies may also interfere with nerve regeneration. In AMAN, axonal damage can result in axonal degeneration (A), or rapid resolution of conduction block (B) (Figure 16).

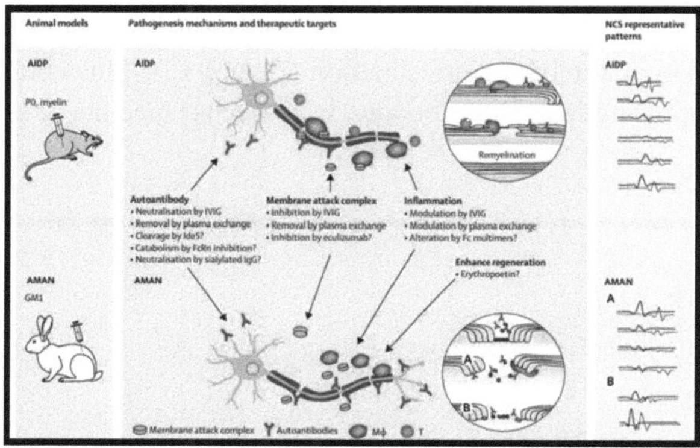

Figure 16: Overview of the pathogenesis and therapeutic targets of two main subtypes of Guillain-Barré syndrome, AIDP and AMAN.

GBS is preceded in approximately 60% of cases by a bacterial or viral infection within 1 to 4 weeks before the onset of the disease. Several microorganisms have been associated with GBS, including Campylobacter jejuni, Zika virus, and, in 2020, acute respiratory syndrome coronavirus (Table II). These infections cause aberrant immune responses resulting in the production of antibodies against myelin constituents and anti-ganglioside antibodies (34). The most common infectious agent implicated in NAFLD is campylobacter jejuni (23). AIDP is most frequently associated with CMV and EBV infections (35, 36).

Table II: The different agents involved in the occurrence of Guillain-Barré syndrome (23)

Trigger		Frequency
Bacteria		
	Campylobacter jejuni	+++
	Mycoplamsa pneumoniae	++
	Hemophilus influenza	+
	Erlichia chaffeenensis	+
	Orientia tsutsugamushi	+
	Escherichia coli	+
Viruses		
	Cytomegaly	+++
	Zika	+++
	SARS-CoV-2	+++

CHAPTER 3: CONTRIBUTION OF ELECTRONEUROMYOGRAPHY IN CASE OF CLINICAL SUSPICION OF GUILLAIN BARRE SYNDROME

The electroneuromyogram (ENMG) is a complementary examination to the clinical examination of the peripheral nervous system. It is a functional exploration because it allows the evaluation of nerve and muscle function (Figure 17).Neurography allows for a separate study of the sensory and motor nerves, which is important for the exploration of several pathologies including Guillain-Barré syndrome.

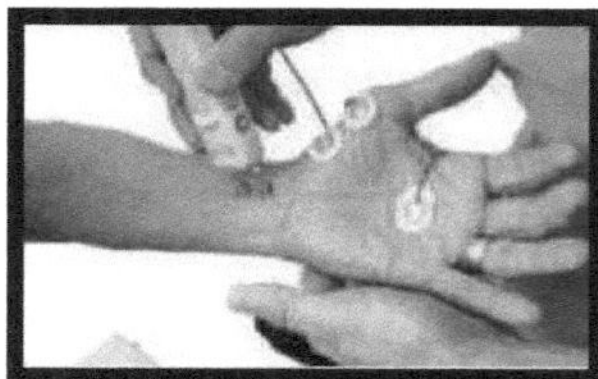

Figure 17: Motor nerve conduction study of the left median nerve

The electrical activity passes from the nerve to the muscle. It can be recorded by surface electrodes (Figure 18). The recorded response is a compound muscle action potential (CMAP).

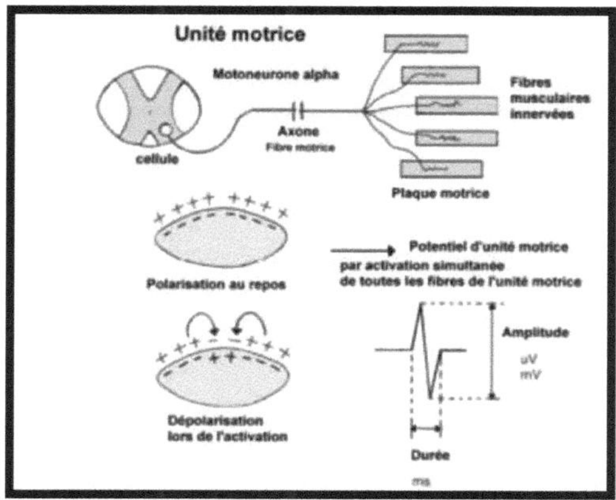

Figure 18: Recording of the motor unit potential

1. STUDY OF MOTOR NERVE CONDUCTION

The study of motor nerve conduction is done by stimulating a point distal and a proximal point on the path of a sought-after nerve (Figure 19).

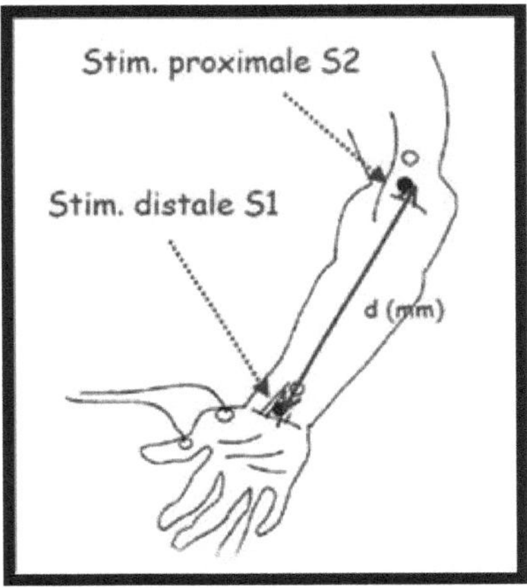

Figure 19: Stimulation points for median nerve motor conduction studies

The different motor nerve conduction parameters studied are the distal motor area, the proximal motor area, the distal motor latency and the motor conduction velocity (Figure 20).

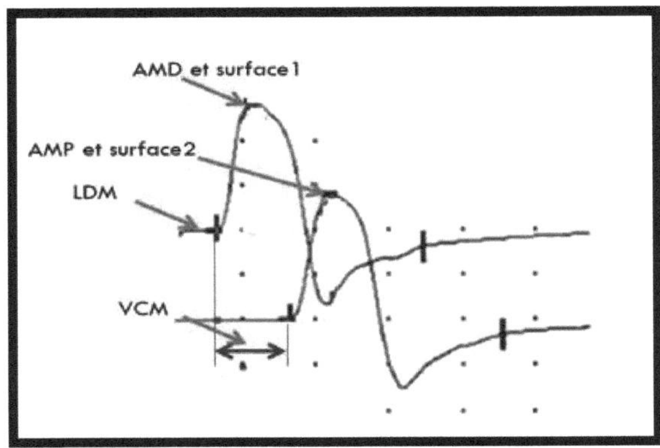

Figure 20: The different parameters of motor nerve conduction

DMA: distal motor area, PMA: proximal motor area, DML: distal motor latency, MCV: motor conduction velocity

***Definition of conduction block:**

It is a decrease in the amplitudes and surfaces of the responses of more of 20%. A conduction block (CB) is likely if the decrease is 20 to 30%. If this decrease is >30%, we speak of definite BC (except for the external popliteal sciatic nerve, a decrease >50% is required) (Figure 21).

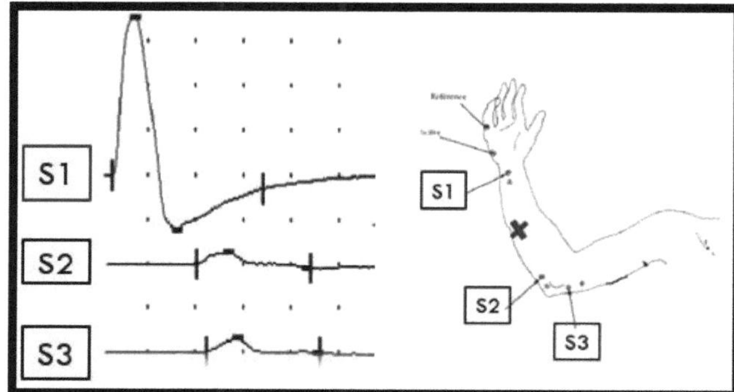

Figure 21: Motor conduction block of the right ulnar nerve at the level of the forearm

It is important to differentiate between a temporal dispersion and a BC (Figure 22). Indeed, a reduction in area <20% with a decrease in amplitude > 20% reflects a temporal dispersion and not a BC.

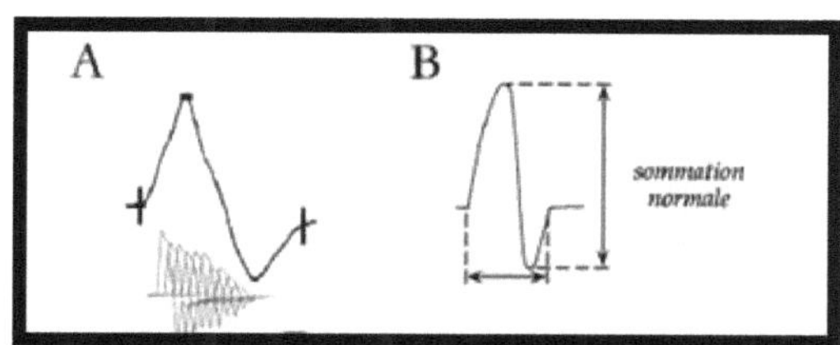

Normal response

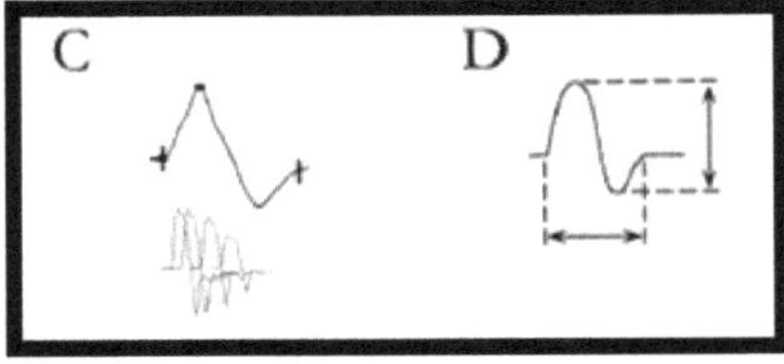

Conduction block

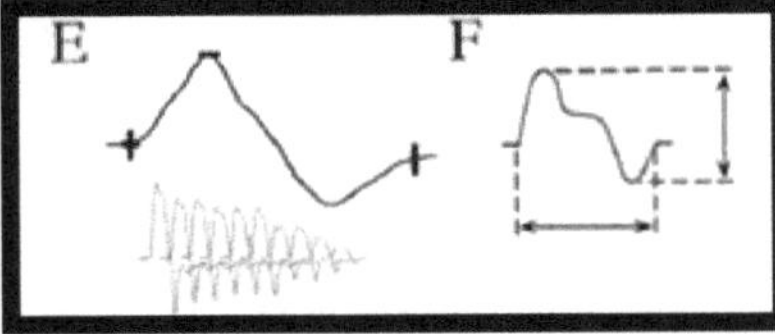

Time dispersion

Figure 22: Differentiating between time dispersion and conduction block

2. STUDY OF WAVES PARAMETERS OF PROXIMAL CONDUCTION

2.1. F-wave

The F-wave is an antidromic discharge of one (or 2) motor units (Figure 23). It appears in supramaximal stimulation. It is a polymorphic wave and in electroneurography, we are mainly interested in its minimal latency.

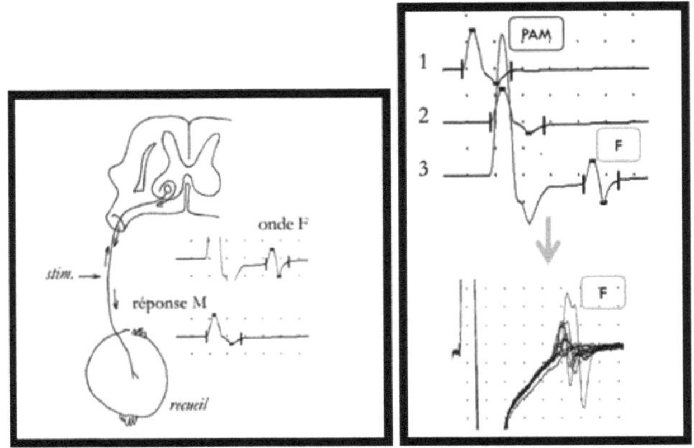

Figure 23: Study parameters of the F wave

25

MAP: motor action potential

2.2. Reflex H

It appears at low intensity and disappears at high intensity. It is of constant shape and latency (figure 24).

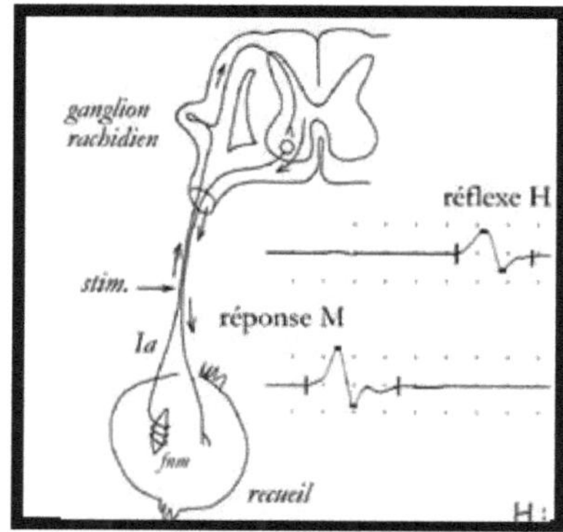

Figure 24: Diagram of the H

3. STUDY OF SENSITIVE NERVE CONDUCTION

The parameters studied are mainly the amplitude and the speed of sensitive conduction (Figure 25).

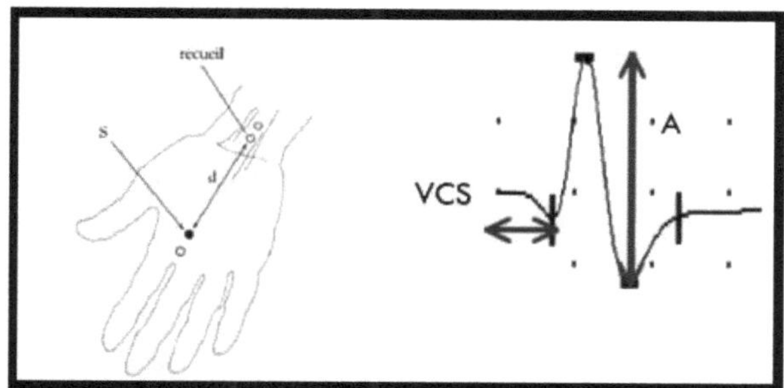

Figure 25: Transcanal sensory conduction study of the right median nerve

*A minimum of 3 sensory and 3 motor nerves with proximal F-wave latency study and bilateral tibial H-reflexes should be performed if GBS is suspected (37).The spectrum of GBS has broadened since its first description in 1916 and is currently used to refer to a range of acute autoimmune neuropathies with different clinical phenotypes.Several diagnostic criteria have been proposed for classical GBS and its relatives(38, 39).There are several electrophysiological variants of GBS with different prognoses. Indeed, GBS includes demyelinating forms (acute inflammatory demyelinating polyneuropathy "AIDP") and axonal forms (acute motor axonal neuropathy "AMAN" and acute motor sensory axonal neuropathy"AMSAN") (38, 39).The different forms of GBS cannot be distinguished either on clinical manifestations or on therapeutic response, and there are no specific biomarkers(19). The individualization of these forms is based on ENMG criteria and electrophysiological evaluations which play a role determining in the positive diagnosis of GBS, in its classification into its different subtypes and in the prognostic evaluation (17).

The classification of GBS into its different subtypes has repercussions on the prognosis and consequently on the management, the rhythm of clinical and electrical monitoring. An adequate classification is also necessary for a possible involvement in clinical trials. Demyelinating forms are characterized by slowed conduction velocities, conduction blocks (CB) and temporal dispersion, whereas axonal forms are characterized by axonal degeneration causing a decrease in muscle action potential amplitude (MAP).Recently, isolated transient conduction blocks without temporal dispersion have been demonstrated in axonal forms. These transient blocks, due to nodal dysfunction without axonal degeneration, may mimic demyelination, making the classification of the different subtypes more difficult(17, 20). Indeed, the difficult distinction between demyelinating and reversible BC is at the origin of 38% of misclassifications.Several electrophysiological criteria aimed at having an early and accurate classification have been proposed: the Hadden criteria of 1998, the Rajabally criteria in 2015, and the Uncini criteria of 2017(17, 20). These require repeated neurophysiological assessments. These different classifications have different sensitivities and specificities. Few studies have focused on evaluating these criteria in pediatric populations especially since GBS is rare in childhood. The ENMG plays a crucial role in the positive diagnosis, determination of the underlying pathophysiological mechanisms and prognosis of GBS(40). Despite the contribution of electrophysiological explorations, there are still difficulties in adequately classifying GBS into its different subtypes. These difficulties are due to several factors:

1. PIDD can be complicated by axonal degeneration secondary

2. Axonal forms can be manifested electrophysiologically by reversible conduction blocks that can distort the classification

3. The detection of antiganglioside antibodies, known to be markers of the axonal forms, in the AIDP.

Several ENMG criteria have been proposed to distinguish the demyelinating form (AIDP) from the axonal forms (AMAN and AMSAN) (19, 41). The criteria established for AIDP varied according to the threshold values of demyelination and the number of abnormalities necessary to retain the demyelinating subtype. These criteria showed different sensitivities and specificities. The diagnosis of axonal forms was based solely on a pattern of axonal degeneration(29). The criteria of Ho et al proposed in 1995, and revised by Hadden et al in 1998 are the most used. In 2012, Uncini et al noted that in addition to axonal degeneration, reversible conduction blocks, recognized by repeated recordings, enter into the pathophysiology of AMAN. These transient conduction blocks were not recognized in the electrophysiological criteria used and could lead to subtype misdiagnosis. They concluded that these criteria lacked specificity and needed to be updated(17). Rapid recovery can occur when the conduction defect corrects before the development of any axonal degeneration(42). Therefore, a rapid recovery time would be in favor of AMAN with reversible blocks and could be an additional element in favor of the axonal form. The criteria for Rajabally et al in 2015 (19) were proposed to improve the diagnostic specificity of GBS subtypes by a single ENMG study. To define demyelination the criteria and limitations used by Rajabally et al were the basis of the criteria used for the diagnosis of chronic polyradiculonevritis and proved their specificity in distinguishing demyelinating from axonal forms. These criteria were also based on recent data on axonal forms of GBS(41). The exclusive presence of BCs, the association of a single BC with a low PGAM amplitude, or the absence of the F wave in two or more nerves are indicators of an axonal form. In the series of 365 patients by Rajabally et al, the successive use of the 2 classifications of Hadden and Rajabally allowed a transfer of 21% of the patients initially classified as AIDP and 22.2% with equivocal results to the axonal group. No patient was reclassified from the axonal group to the AIDP or equivocal groups. The number of patients with axonal form increased from 17.5% to 35.1%. There was a correlation between the change in subtype and the time to perform ENMG, and patients who were reclassified to the axonal group had ENMG within 7 days of the onset of symptoms (19). In another similar and more recent study by Hiew et al (43) and applying the criteria of Hadden et al and the criteria of Rajabally et al, the percentage of the AMAN form increased from 55% to 67% with a reduction in the percentage of the AIDP form from 29% to 19%. The number of patients with normal or equivocal results remained unchanged.In order to determine whether the criteria of Rajabally et al on the basis of a single ENMG study give similar results to those obtained after serial studies on the same patient population, Uncini et al (19) reanalyzed the data of 55 GBS patients who had serial ENMGs. According to the result of the 1er ENMG there were differences in classifications with according to Hadden 67% AIDP (vs 45% according to Rajabally), 18% axonal (vs 35% according to Rajabally) and 15% equivocal (vs 20% according to Rajabally). After repeat ENMG, the same proportion of patients (24%) changed shape in the 2 classifications, but the relative changes between groups differed. Nine patients (7 equivocal and 2 axonal) according to Rajabally and reclassified as AIDP after serial studies had no antiganglioside antibodies, whereas 4 patients (2 equivocal and 2 AIDP) according to Rajabally reclassified as axonal form had antiganglioside antibodies. The results of this study suggest that serial studies remain the gold standard for the diagnosis of different forms of GBS. However, the Rajabally classification improved the diagnostic sensitivity and specificity after a single evaluation.For AMAN, the sensitivity was 81% and specificity 94% when applying Rajabally's criteria, compared with a sensitivity of 47% and specificity of 100% found with Hadden's criteria on repeated EMGs. This increase in sensitivity was due to the introduction of conduction blocks as a parameter for the diagnosis of the axonal form of GBS. BCs were considered an expression of segmental demyelination, when saltatory conduction stops and the axon remains intact(44). Recently, transient, reversible BCs secondary to the binding of anti-ganglioside antibodies to the nodes of Ranvier have been shown to interrupt nerve conduction without associated axonal degeneration(45, 46). For the AIDP, the sensitivity was 70% and the specificity 96% compared to a sensitivity of 94% and a specificity of 72% found with the Hadden criteria. This increase in specificity could be explained by the more stringent criteria for demyelination used by Rajabally and colleagues(33). These criteria have indeed proven their specificity in chronic polyradiculonevritis. An important limitation of Rajabally's criteria is that they do not take into account the existence of a possible temporal dispersion. This temporal dispersion, which translates into a lengthening of the duration of the muscle action potential (asynchronous conduction at the level of the nerve fibers), is a characteristic of remyelination, which follows the demyelination process and makes it possible to distinguish between axonal and demyelinating forms(33). Uncini et al suggest in their new criteria project to take into account this temporal dispersion which is a better criterion of demyelination than conduction blocks. They use serial ENMGs to differentiate reversible transient BC from axonal degeneration at $2^{\text{ème}}$ ENMGs (33, 47).

•Limitations of the ENMG:

*When studying motor nerve conduction, a conduction block distal (Figure 26) may mimic axonal loss.

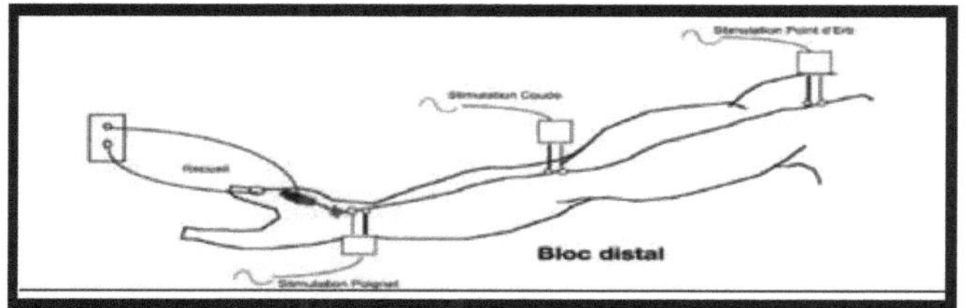

Figure 26: Distal conduction block of the left median nerve

*a very proximal motor nerve conduction block (Figure 27) may be associated with normal motor conductance, despite an obvious motor deficit

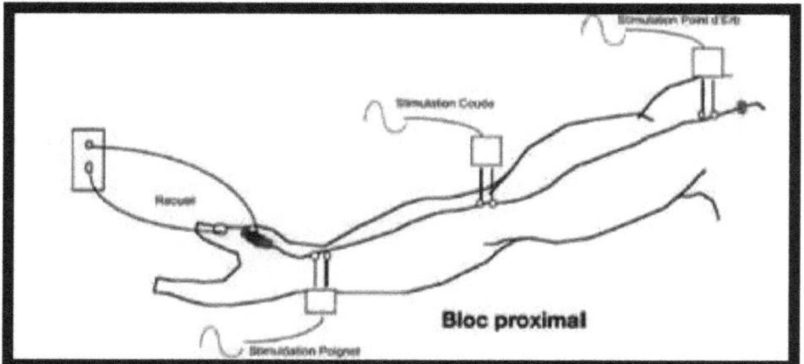

Figure 27: Proximal conduction block of the left median nerve

* When detected, fibrillation does not occur until 10 to 15 days after nerve destruction.

* Abnormalities suggestive of demyelination may occur very early but are **non-specific.** They will only be convincing after the third week.

* A positive diagnosis and certain prognosis would only be possible on an ENMG of the 3rd or 4th week^{ème}

BIBLIOGRAPHY

1.Farley A, Johnstone C, Hendry C, McLafferty E. Nervous system: part 1. Nursing standard (Royal College of Nursing (Great Britain): 1987. 2014;28(31):46-51.

2.Mohassel P, Chaudhry V. Neurophysiology simplified for imagers. Seminars in musculoskeletal radiology. 2015;19(2):112-20.

3.Wehrwein EA, Orer HS, Barman SM. Overview of the Anatomy, Physiology, and Pharmacology of the Autonomic Nervous System. Comprehensive Physiology. 2016;6(3):1239-78.

4.Rigoard P, Buffenoir K, Wager M, Bauche S, Giot JP, Robert R, et al [Anatomy and physiology of the peripheral nerve]. Neuro-Chirurgie. 2009;55 Suppl 1:S3-12.

5.Catala M, Kubis N. Gross anatomy and development of the peripheral nervous system. Handbook of clinical neurology. 2013;115:29-41.

6.Hendry C, Farley A, McLafferty E, Johnstone C. Nervous system: part 2. Nursing standard (Royal College of Nursing (Great Britain): 1987). 2014;28(32):45-9.

7.Farley A, McLafferty E, Johnstone C, Hendry C. Nervous system: part 3. Nursing standard (Royal College of Nursing (Great Britain): 1987). 2014;28(33):46-50.

8.Sheikh KA. Guillain-Barré Syndrome. Continuum (Minneapolis, Minn). 2020;26(5):1184-204.

9.Marcus R. What Is Guillain-Barré Syndrome? Jama. 2023.
10. Mirian A, Nicolle MW, Budhram A. Guillain-Barré syndrome. CMAJ: Canadian Medical Association journal = journal de l'Association medicale canadienne. 2021;193(11):E378.

11. Florian IA, Lupan I, Sur L, Samasca G, Timiş TL. To be, or not to be... Guillain-Barré Syndrome. Autoimmunity reviews. 2021;20(12):102983.
12. Chakraborty T, Kramer CL, Wijdicks EFM, Rabinstein AA. Dysautonomia in Guillain-Barré Syndrome: Prevalence, Clinical Spectrum, and Outcomes. Neurocritical care. 2020;32(1):113-20.

13. Shahrizaila N, Lehmann HC, Kuwabara S. Guillain-Barré syndrome. Lancet (London, England). 2021;397(10280):1214-28.

14. Nguyen TP, Taylor RS. Guillain Barre Syndrome. StatPearls. Treasure Island, FL: StatPearls Publishing. Copyright © 2022, StatPearls Publishing LLC; 2022.

15. McGrogan A, Madle GC, Seaman HE, de Vries CS. The epidemiology of Guillain-Barré syndrome worldwide. A systematic literature review. Neuroepidemiology. 2009;32(2):150-63.

16. Roodbol J, de Wit MC, Aarsen FK, Catsman-Berrevoets CE, Jacobs BC. Long-term outcome of Guillain-Barré syndrome in children. Journal of the peripheral nervous system: JPNS. 2014;19(2):121-6.

17. Uncini A, Kuwabara S. Electrodiagnostic criteria for Guillain-Barrè syndrome: a critical revision and the need for an update. Clinical neurophysiology: official journal of the International Federation of Clinical Neurophysiology. 2012;123(8):1487-95.

18. Devos D, Magot A, Perrier-Boeswillwald J, Fayet G, Leclair-Visonneau L, Ollivier Y, et al. Guillain-Barré syndrome during childhood: particular clinical and electrophysiological features. Muscle & nerve. 2013;48(2):247- 51.

19. Rajabally YA, Durand MC, Mitchell J, Orlikowski D, Nicolas G. Electrophysiological diagnosis of Guillain-Barré syndrome subtype: could a single study suffice? Journal of neurology, neurosurgery, and psychiatry. 2015;86(1):115-9.

20. Uncini A, Ippoliti L, Shahrizaila N, Sekiguchi Y, Kuwabara S. Optimizing the electrodiagnostic accuracy in Guillain-Barré syndrome subtypes: Criteria sets and sparse linear discriminant analysis. Clinical neurophysiology : official journal of the International Federation of Clinical Neurophysiology. 2017;128(7):1176-83.

21. Fokke C, van den Berg B, Drenthen J, Walgaard C, van Doorn PA, Jacobs BC. Diagnosis of Guillain-Barré syndrome and validation of Brighton criteria. Brain: a journal of neurology. 2014;137(Pt 1):33-43.

22. Korinthenberg R, Trollmann R, Felderhoff-Müser U, Bernert G, Hackenberg A, Hufnagel M, et al. Diagnosis and treatment of Guillain-Barré Syndrome in childhood and adolescence: An evidence- and consensus-based guideline. European journal of paediatric neurology : EJPN : official journal of the

European Paediatric Neurology Society. 2020;25:5-16.

23. Finsterer J. Triggers of Guillain-Barré Syndrome: Campylobacter jejuni Predominates. International journal of molecular sciences. 2022;23(22).

24. Bickerstaff ER. Brain-stem encephalitis; further observations on a grave syndrome with benign prognosis. British medical journal. 1957;1(5032):1384- 7.

25. Carpentier VT, Le Guennec L, Fall SAA, Viala K, Demeret S, Weiss N. [Pathophysiological and diagnostic aspects of Guillain-Barré syndrome]. La Revue de medecine interne. 2022;43(7):419-28.

26. Ropper AH. Further regional variants of acute immune polyneuropathy. Bifacial weakness or sixth nerve paresis with paresthesias, lumbar polyradiculopathy, and ataxia with pharyngeal-cervical-brachial weakness. Archives of neurology. 1994;51(7):671-5.

27. Mericle RA, Triggs WJ. Treatment of acute pandysautonomia with intravenous immunoglobulin. Journal of neurology, neurosurgery, and psychiatry. 1997;62(5):529-31.

28. Payus AO, Ibrahim A, Liew Sat Lin C, Hui Jan T. Sensory Predominant Guillain-Barré Syndrome Concomitant with Dengue Infection: A Case Report. Case reports in neurology. 2022;14(2):281-5.

29. Dash S, Pai AR, Kamath U, Rao P. Pathophysiology and diagnosis of Guillain-Barré syndrome - challenges and needs. The international journal of neuroscience. 2015;125(4):235-40.

30. Yuki N, Hartung HP. Guillain-Barré syndrome. The New England journal of medicine. 2012;366(24):2294-304.

31. Hiraga A, Mori M, Ogawara K, Hattori T, Kuwabara S. Differences in patterns of progression in demyelinating and axonal Guillain-Barré syndromes. Neurology. 2003;61(4):471-4.

32. Sekiguchi Y, Uncini A, Yuki N, Misawa S, Notturno F, Nasu S, et al. Antiganglioside antibodies are associated with axonal Guillain-Barré syndrome: a Japanese-Italian collaborative study. Journal of neurology, neurosurgery, and psychiatry. 2012;83(1):23-8.

33. Uncini A, Zappasodi F, Notturno F. Electrodiagnosis of GBS subtypes by a single study: not yet the squaring of the circle. Journal of neurology, neurosurgery, and psychiatry. 2015;86(1):5-8.

34. Laman JD, Huizinga R, Boons GJ, Jacobs BC. Guillain-Barré syndrome: expanding the concept of molecular mimicry. Trends in immunology. 2022;43(4):296-308.

35. Ogawara K, Kuwabara S, Mori M, Hattori T, Koga M, Yuki N. Axonal Guillain-Barré syndrome: relation to anti-ganglioside antibodies and Campylobacter jejuni infection in Japan. Annals of neurology. 2000;48(4):624-31.

36. van Koningsveld R, Schmitz PI, Meché FG, Visser LH, Meulstee J, van Doorn PA. Effect of methylprednisolone when added to standard treatment with intravenous immunoglobulin for Guillain-Barré syndrome: randomised trial. Lancet (London, England). 2004;363(9404):192-6.

37. Hughes RA, Cornblath DR. Guillain-Barré syndrome. Lancet (London, England). 2005;366(9497):1653-66.

38. Wakerley BR, Uncini A, Yuki N. Guillain-Barré and Miller Fisher syndromes--new diagnostic classification. Nature reviews Neurology. 2014;10(9):537-44.

39. McKhann GM, Cornblath DR, Griffin JW, Ho TW, Li CY, Jiang Z, et al. Acute motor axonal neuropathy: a frequent cause of acute flaccid paralysis in China. Annals of neurology. 1993;33(4):333-42.

40. Uncini A, Manzoli C, Notturno F, Capasso M. Pitfalls in electrodiagnosis of Guillain-Barré syndrome subtypes. Journal of neurology, neurosurgery, and psychiatry. 2010;81(10):1157-63.

41. Van den Bergh PY, Piéret F. Electrodiagnostic criteria for acute and chronic inflammatory demyelinating polyradiculoneuropathy. Muscle & nerve. 2004;29(4):565-74.

42. Capasso M, Caporale CM, Pomilio F, Gandolfi P, Lugaresi A, Uncini A. Acute motor conduction block neuropathy Another Guillain-Barré syndrome variant. Neurology. 2003;61(5):617-22.

43. Hiew FL, Ramlan R, Viswanathan S, Puvanarajah S. Guillain-Barré syndrome, variants & fruste forms: Reclassification with new criteria. Clinical neurology and neurosurgery. 2017;158:114-8.

44. Kokubun N, Nishibayashi M, Uncini A, Odaka M, Hirata K, Yuki N. Conduction block in acute motor axonal neuropathy. Brain: a journal of

neurology. 2010;133(10):2897-908.

45. Susuki K, Yuki N, Schafer DP, Hirata K, Zhang G, Funakoshi K, et al. Dysfunction of nodes of Ranvier: a mechanism for anti-ganglioside antibody-mediated neuropathies. Experimental neurology. 2011;233(1):534-42.

46. Uncini A, Susuki K, Yuki N. Nodo-paranodopathy: beyond the demyelinating and axonal classification in anti-ganglioside antibody-mediated neuropathies. Clinical neurophysiology : official journal of the International Federation of Clinical Neurophysiology. 2013;124(10):1928-34.

47. Uncini A, Kuwabara S. The electrodiagnosis of Guillain-Barré syndrome subtypes: Where do we stand? Clinical neurophysiology : official journal of the International Federation of Clinical Neurophysiology. 2018;129(12):2586- 93.

APPENDIX 1: DIAGNOSTIC CRITERIA FOR THE CLASSIC FORM OF GBS WAKERLEY ET AL 2014

Classification	Core clinical features	Notes	Supportive features
General syndrome			
All GBS spectrum disorders	Mostly symmetric pattern of limb and/or motor cranial-nerve weakness*[§] Monophasic disease course with interval between onset and nadir of weakness of 12h to 28 days, followed by clinical plateau	Alternative diagnosis should be excluded	Antecedent infectious symptoms[¶] Presence of distal paraesthesia at or before the onset of weakness Cerebrospinal fluid albuminocytological dissociation[†]
Specific diagnoses			
Classic GBS	Weakness* and areflexia/ hyporeflexia in all four limbs	Weakness usually starts in the legs and ascends but may start in the arms Weakness may be mild, moderate or complete paralysis Cranial-nerve-innervated muscles or respiratory muscles may be involved Muscle stretch reflexes may be normal or exaggerated in 10% of cases	Electrophysiological evidence of neuropathy

APPENDIX 2: HADDEN ET AL 1998 CRITERIA

Box 1 Hadden *et al*'s electrodiagnostic criteria for Guillain–Barré syndrome

1. Normal
   (All the following in all nerves tested)
   - DML ≤100% ULN
   - F-wave present with latency ≤100% ULN
   - MCV ≥100% LLN
   - Distal CMAP ≥100% LLN
   - Proximal CMAP ≥100% LLN
   - Proximal CMAP/distal CMAP ratio >0.5
2. Primary demyelinating
   (At least one of the following in each of at least two nerves, or at least two of the following in one nerve if all others inexcitable and distal CMAP ≥10% LLN)
   - MCV <90% LLN (85% if Distal CMAP <50% LLN)
   - DML >110% ULN (120% if Distal CMAP <100% LLN)
   - Proximal CMAP/distal CMAP ratio <0.5 and distal CMAP ≥20% LLN
   - F-response latency >120% ULN
3. Primary axonal
   - None of the above features of demyelination in any nerve (except one demyelinating feature allowed in one nerve if distal CMAP <10% LLN) and
   - Distal CMAP <80% LLN in at least two nerves
4. Inexcitable
   - Distal CMAP absent in all nerves (or present in only one nerve with distal CMAP <10% LLN)
5. Equivocal
   - Does not exactly fit criteria for any other group

CMAP, compound muscle action potentials; DML, distal motor latency; LLN, lower limit of normal; MCV, motor conduction velocity; ULN, upper limit of normal.

APPENDIX 3: RAJABALLY ET AL 2015 CRITERIA.

criteria for Guillain–Barré syndrome (based on Van den Bergh and Piéret, for demyelinating cut-offs and incorporating use of new knowledge on axonal GBS to define primary axonal forms)

1. Normal
   (All the following in all nerves tested)
   - DML ≤100% ULN
   - F-wave present with latency ≤100% ULN
   - MCV ≥100% LLN
   - Distal CMAP ≥100% LLN
   - Proximal CMAP/distal CMAP ratio >0.7 (excluding the tibial nerve)
2. Acute inflammatory demyelinating polyradiculoneuropathy (AIDP)
   - At least one of the following in at least two nerves:
     - MCV <70% LLN
     - DML >150% ULN
     - F-response latency >120% ULN, or >150% ULN (if distal CMAP <50% of LLN)
   - OR
     - F-wave absence in two nerves with distal CMAP ≥20% LLN, with an additional parameter, in one other nerve
   - OR
     - Proximal CMAP/distal CMAP ratio <0.7 (excluding the tibial nerve), in two nerves with an additional parameter, in one other nerve
3. Axonal GBS including inexcitable forms
   - *Axonal GBS:*
   None of the above features of demyelination in any nerve (except one demyelinating feature allowed in one nerve if distal CMAP <10% LLN), and at least one of the following:
     - Distal CMAP <80% LLN in two nerves
     - F-wave absence in two nerves with distal CMAP ≥20% LLN, in absence of any demyelinating feature in any nerve
     - Proximal CMAP/distal CMAP ratio <0.7, in two nerves (excluding the tibial nerve)
     - F-wave absence in one nerve with distal CMAP ≥20% LLN OR proximal CMAP/distal CMAP ratio <0.7 (excluding the tibial nerve), in one nerve; with IN ADDITION, distal CMAP <80% LLN in one other nerve
   - Inexcitable:
   If distal CMAP absent in all nerves (or present in only one nerve with distal CMAP <10% LLN)
4. Equivocal
   - Abnormal range findings however not fitting criteria for any other group

CMAP, compound muscle action potentials; DML, distal motor latency; GBS, Guillain–Barré syndrome; LLN, lower limit of normal; MCV, motor conduction velocity; ULN, upper limit of normal.

APPENDIX 4: UNCINI CRITERIA AND AL 2017

1) Acute inflammatory demyelinating polyneuropathy (AIDP)

At first or second study at least one of the following in at least two nerves:

- MCV <70% LLN
- DML >130 % ULN
- dCMAP duration >120% ULN
- pCMAP/dCMAP duration >130%
- F-response latency >120% ULN
  OR one of the above in one nerve PLUS:
- Absent F waves in two nerves with dCMAP >20% LLN
- Abnormal ulnar SNAP amplitude and normal sural SNAP amplitude

2) Axonal GBS

Acute motor axonal neuropathy (AMAN)

At first and second study none of the above AIDP features in any nerve (demyelinating features allowed in one nerve if dCMAP <20% LLN)

At first study at least one of the following in each of two nerves:

- dCMAP < 80% LLN
- pCMAP/dCMAP amplitude ratio < 0.7 (excluding tibial nerve)
- isolated F wave absence (or < 20% persistence)

At second study:

at least one of the followings in two nerves is evidence of axonal degeneration:

- persistent or further reduction of dCMAP amplitude
- pCMAP/dCMAP amplitude ratio < 0.7 at first test which recovers because of decrease of dCMAP without increased temporal dispersion (dCMAP duration $\leq$ 120% ULN and pCMAP/dCMAP duration ratio $\leq$ 130%)

at least one of the followings in two nerves is evidence of reversible conduction failure:

- >150% increase dCMAP amplitude without increased dCMAP duration ($\leq$120% ULN)
- pCMAP/dCMAP amplitude ratio <0.7 at first test which improves more than 0.2 because of increased pCMAP without temporal dispersion (pCMAP/d CMAP duration ratio $\leq$ 130%)
- isolated F wave absence (or <20% persistence) that recovers without increased minimal latency ($\leq$120% of ULN)

Acute motor and sensory axonal neuropathy (AMSAN)

At first study

- the same criteria of AMAN in motor nerves
  PLUS
- SNAP amplitudes <50%LLN in at least two nerves

At second study:

- evidence for axonal degeneration and reversible conduction failure in motor nerves as in AMAN
- **there is evidence of axonal degeneration in sensory nerves** if SNAP amplitude in two nerves it is stable or decreased
- **there is evidence of reversible conduction failure in sensory nerves** if SNAP amplitude in two nerves it is increased (>50% in median and ulnar nerves and >60% in sural)

3) Inexcitable

At first or second study

- Distal CMAP absent in all nerves (or present in only one with distal CMAP <10% LLN)

4) Equivocal

At first or second study

- Abnormal findings not fulfilling any of the above criteria

APPENDIX 5: ELECTRICAL CRITERIA FOR THE DIAGNOSIS OF GUILLAIN-BARRE SYNDROME

Table 1

Electrodiagnostic criteria sets for Guillain-Barré syndrome by Hadden et al. (1998), Rajabally et al. (2015) and Uncini et al. (2017).

Hadden's criteria	Rajabally's criteria	Uncini's criteria
1) Primary demyelinating At least one of the following in each of two nerves, or at least two of the following in one nerve if all others inexcitable and distal CMAP ≥10% LLN • MCV <90% LLN (85% if dCMAP <50% LLN) • DML >110% ULN (120% if dCMAP <100% LLN) • pCMAP/dCMAP amplitude ratio <0.5 and distal CMAP ≥20% LLN • F-response latency >120% ULN **2) Primary axonal** • None of the above features of demyelination in any nerve (except one demyelinating feature allowed in one nerve if distal CMAP <10% LLN AND • dCMAP <80% LLN in at least two nerves **3) Inexcitable** • dCMAP absent in all nerves (or present in only one nerve with distal CMAP <10% LLN) **4) Equivocal** • Does not exactly fit criteria for any other group	**1) Acute inflammatory demyelinating polyneuropathy (AIDP)** At least one of the following in at least two nerves: • MCV <70% LLN • DML >150% ULN • F-response latency >120% ULN, or >150% ULN (if distal CMAP <50% of LLN) OR • F-wave absence in two nerves with dCMAP ≥20% LLN, with an additional parameter, in one other nerve OR • pCMAP/dCMAP amplitude ratio <0.7 (excluding the tibial nerve), in two nerves with an additional parameter, in one other nerve **2) Axonal GBS (including inexcitable forms)** **Axonal GBS** None of the above features of demyelination in any nerve (except one demyelinating feature allowed in one nerve if dCMAP <10% LLN), and at least one of the following: • dCMAP <80% LLN in two nerves • F-wave absence in two nerves with distal CMAP ≥20% LLN, in absence of any demyelinating feature in any nerve • pCMAP/dCMAP amplitude ratio <0.7, in two nerves (excluding the tibial nerve) • F-wave absence in one nerve with distal CMAP ≥20% LLN OR pCMAP/d CMAP amplitude ratio <0.7 (excluding the tibial nerve), in one nerve; with **IN ADDITION**, dCMAP <80% LLN in one other nerve **Inexcitable** • If dCMAP absent in all nerves (or present in only one nerve with dCMAP <10% LLN) **3) Equivocal** • Abnormal range findings however not fitting criteria for any other group	**1) Acute inflammatory demyelinating polyneuropathy (AIDP)** *At first or second study* at least one of the following in at least two nerves: • MCV <70% LLN • DML >130 % ULN • dCMAP duration >120% ULN • pCMAP/dCMAP duration >130% • F-response latency >120% ULN **OR one of the above in one nerve PLUS:** • Absent F waves in two nerves with dCMAP >20% LLN • Abnormal ulnar SNAP amplitude and normal sural SNAP amplitude **2) Axonal GBS** Acute motor axonal neuropathy (AMAN) *At first and second study* none of the above AIDP features in any nerve (demyelinating features allowed in one nerve if dCMAP <20% LLN) *At first study* at least one of the following in each of two nerves: • dCMAP < 80% LLN • pCMAP/dCMAP amplitude ratio < 0.7 (excluding tibial nerve) • isolated F wave absence (or < 20% persistence) *At second study:* **at least one of the followings in two nerves is evidence of axonal degeneration:** • persistent or further reduction of dCMAP amplitude • pCMAP/dCMAP amplitude ratio < 0.7 at first test which recovers because of decrease of dCMAP without increased temporal dispersion (dCMAP duration ≤ 120% ULN and pCMAP/dCMAP duration ratio ≤ 130%) **at least one of the followings in two nerves is evidence of reversible conduction failure:** • >150% increase dCMAP amplitude without increased dCMAP duration (≤120% ULN) • pCMAP/dCMAP amplitude ratio <0.7 at first test which improves more than 0.2 because of increased pCMAP without temporal dispersion (pCMAP/d CMAP duration ratio ≤ 130%) • isolated F wave absence (or <20% persistence) that recovers without increased minimal latency (≤120% of ULN) **Acute motor and sensory axonal neuropathy (AMSAN)** *At first study* • the same criteria of AMAN in motor nerves **PLUS** • SNAP amplitudes <50%LLN in at least two nerves *At second study:* • evidence for axonal degeneration and reversible conduction failure in motor nerves as in AMAN • **there is evidence of axonal degeneration in sensory nerves** if SNAP amplitude in two nerves it is stable or decreased • **there is evidence of reversible conduction failure in sensory nerves** if SNAP amplitude in two nerves it is increased (>50% in median and ulnar nerves and >60% in sural) **3) Inexcitable** *At first or second study* • Distal CMAP absent in all nerves (or present in only one with distal CMAP <10% LLN) **4) Equivocal** *At first or second study* • Abnormal findings not fulfilling any of the above criteria

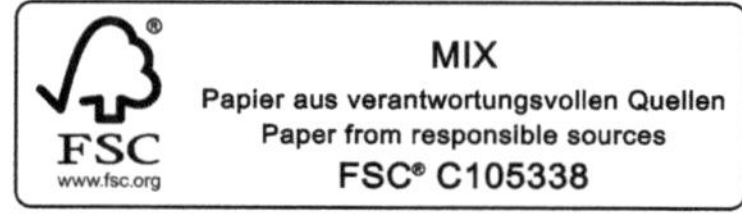

Printed by Books on Demand GmbH, Norderstedt / Germany